Alkaline Diet

How to Improve Your Health and Balance Your PH with the Power of the Alkaline Diet, including Alkaline Foods and Alkaline Recipes

Copyright 2015

Table Of Contents

Introduction 1

Chapter 1:   Introduction to the Alkaline Diet 2

Chapter 2:   Alkaline Foods 7

Chapter 3:   Breakfast 15

Chapter 4:   Soups and Stews 24

Chapter 5:   Salads 31

Chapter 6:   Entrees 43

Conclusion 51

Introduction

I want to thank you and congratulate you for downloading the book, "Alkaline Diet".

This book contains helpful information about the alkaline diet, how it works, and how you can use it to improve your health.

The alkaline diet aims to balance the PH levels of your body to a more stable, alkaline, level. Most people are too acidic, and this can lead to a range of health problems and feelings of lethargy.

Through using the alkaline diet, you will be able to improve your overall health, stay safe from diseases and illnesses, and experience more energy and vitality!

This book will explain to you tips and techniques that will allow you to begin successfully implementing the alkaline diet into your own life, and reaping the health benefits that it has to offer!

To get you started, this book includes a range of alkaline recipes, including recipes for breakfast, smoothies, entrees, soups, main meals, and more!

Read on to begin improving your health with the power of the alkaline diet, today!

Thanks again for downloading this book, I hope you enjoy it!

Chapter 1:
Introduction to the Alkaline Diet

When you consume more acidifying foods than you do alkalizing foods, an acid ash is developed inside the body. Eating mostly meat, grains, and dairy create a more acidic environment inside the body, which makes it very conducive for bacteria, fungi, and yeasts. The worst part is that the presence of these micro-forms will cause the body to become even more acidic, thus making it highly susceptible to diseases and other health concerns.

The Alkaline diet seeks to create a pH balance inside the body in order to get rid of the excess acid present. Certain minerals in the alkaline diet can neutralize the acids. It is generally recommended that your diet should be made up of about 80 percent of alkalizing foods in order to restore balance.

The Alkaline Diet

The main purpose of the alkaline diet is to balance the natural pH or potential hydrogen ratio of the body. The ideal pH of the body should always fall within the range of 7.33 and 7.4. However, due to the traditionally high acid diet that most people follow, it is highly likely that one should start following the alkaline diet.

Everything that we put inside our bodies releases either an acidic or an alkaline base into the blood. These are then regulated by the blood, saliva, and urine in order to make sure that it is slightly alkaline and falls within the safe pH range that will enable the body to properly function and remain immune from fungal, viral, and bacterial infections.

Whenever the pH in the body gets too acidic, the body will have to resort to stored sources of alkalinity from within itself, such as calcium, magnesium, sodium, and potassium. The first source is always from the bones and teeth, as it contains calcium. The reason why many people suffer from osteoporosis is due to a highly acidic diet. Plaque is caused by an acidic diet as well, and it can be found in the arteries and the teeth.

Acid, upon entering the bloodstream, creates candida or yeast colonies which continue to thrive in an acidic environment. They are primarily found in the digestive tract, then make their way into the bloodstream and become distributed throughout the cells.

If a person continues to follow an acidic diet and does not do anything to restore his or her pH balance, he will eventually suffer from a wide range of complications from tooth decay, fatigue, and a poor immune system to kidney failure, heart disease, liver failure, and other degenerative health issues.

The Benefits of the Alkaline Diet

When a person follows a consistently balanced alkaline diet, he or she will experience feeling more energy, and enjoy immunity against diseases. For instance, our body's energy level depends on its production of adenosine triphosphate or ATP. Only a body with a balanced pH level can produce adequate amounts of this base.

Bacterial growth in the mouth can cause tooth decay and bad breath, so if you are a person who wishes to prevent oral problems or wants to treat any existing issues, then the alkaline diet is highly recommended for you. The alkaline diet discourages the development of bad bacteria, and works to keep you disease and illness free.

The diet is also rich in magnesium, which helps keep the tissues and joints properly functioning and healthy. Cellular repair is also more effective because the body is better able to cleanse out the free radicals or toxins that are built up in the cells. In other words, an alkaline diet can possibly slow down the aging process.

Healthy Alkaline Foods

The alkaline diet is rich in fresh vegetables, legumes, seeds, and nuts. To add flavor to its dishes, the diet makes use of a variety of spices, herbs, and low acid seasonings. Some staple seasonings that are in the alkaline dieter's kitchen are tamari, ginger, miso, cinnamon, curry, chili pepper, and mustard. Sea salt, which has a low pH, is acceptable as well.

Dark green leafy vegetables are among the most alkaline foods out there, such as broccoli, kale, and cucumber. Avocado is a fruit that is touted to have a very high alkaline content, as well as lemons, limes, bananas, and figs. Root vegetables are another source of low pH levels, such as white radishes, turnips, and rutabagas. Sweet potatoes, yams, and potatoes are also a part of this list.

Instead of meat, people who strictly follow the alkaline diet turn to tofu as their main source of protein. Other sources are whey protein powder and tempeh, as well as millet, almonds, and chestnuts. Oils and seeds that contain high alkaline content are olive, coconut, sesame, fennel, and caraway.

Preparing for the Alkaline Diet

It is important to consult your doctor before making any major changes in your diet. People who have acute or chronic kidney failure should not follow a mostly alkaline diet without the approval of a medical professional. This is because the high potassium content can counteract with the medications used for treating kidney problems.

You can also test the pH level in your body by buying the pH test strips from local pharmacies. A sample of your saliva and/or urine is needed to check if you have too much or too little alkalinity.

Certain guidelines should also be followed in order to maximize the alkaline diet:

For instance, fruit should be eaten sparingly as it is processed by the body as a sugar and can contribute to the acidity level in the body. Whenever you wish to eat fruit, you should either eat it alone, cooked, or prior to eating a large meal. Never eat fruit after eating a large meal, as this will cause the fruit to ferment and turn acidic.

Chemical foods such as Splenda, Equal, and all other aspartame should also be avoided as they contribute to an acidic environment as well. If you are required to take antibiotics, ask your doctor if you can take probiotics afterwards to counteract their acidic effects.

In an alkaline diet, you must do whatever it takes to avoid sugar and yeast, as well as fermented and processed food. Yeast feeds on sugar in order to survive in the body, and it will take several weeks of not eating sugar before the yeast subsides. Take care, though, because once you have gotten rid of sugar from your system, the yeast in your body will trigger you to crave for even more of it. It will take discipline to say no to those cravings and eliminate the spread of yeast in your body.

Keep in mind that you may experience symptoms which are a bit similar to the flu when you first start the alkaline diet. Do not worry, for this is just your body withdrawing from the traditional diet that it has gotten used to. After a few days, this will be gone and you will feel even better than you did before.

Once you are ready to plan and prepare for your alkaline diet, it is important to choose meals that offer variety and minimize your consumption of foods that are high in acid, including beef, pork, coffee, peanuts, and processed cheeses. However, you should also include high alkaline foods, such as broccoli, raisins, and spinach, in moderation.

Chapter 2: Alkaline Foods

Once you are ready to start your alkaline diet, keep a list of the following foods in your smartphone or on your refrigerator. That way, you will know what to buy during your next trip to the grocery store and/or farmer's market. Most of these foods are alkaline by nature, and some of them are known to be acidic but actually have alkalizing effects once digested by the body.

Vegetables

- Avocado
- Cucumber
- Leeks
- Beet greens
- Edible gourds
- Peas
- Salad greens
- Broccoli
- Fennel
- Peppers
- Spinach
- Brussels sprouts
- Garlic
- Potato
- Squash
- Carrots
- Wheat-grass
- Radish
- Sweet potatoes
- Celery stalks
- Green beans
- Red beets
- Turnips
- Chives

- Green cabbage
- Red cabbage
- Watercress
- Corn
- Leeks
- Rhubarb
- Yellow beans
- Zucchini
- Artichokes
- Cauliflower
- Lettuce
- Onion
- Peas

Dried Fruits

- Apricots
- Bananas
- Dates
- Raisins

Fresh Fruits

- Coconut
- Sour cherries
- Watermelon
- Lemon
- Lime
- Grapefruit

Beans and Legumes

- Navy beans
- Soy beans

- Soy nuts
- Soy sprouts
- White beans
- Tofu
- Dried peas

- Lentils
- Kidney beans
- Mung beans
- Chickpeas (garbanzo beans)
- Red beans

Cereal Grain

- Buckwheat
- Granola
- Millet
- Oats
- crackers, cereals, pasta, bread (no yeast)

- Quinoa
- Rye
- Whole grain

Dairy Products and Beverages

- Fresh butter
- Fresh buttermilk
- Fresh cheese
- Fresh whey
- Acidophilus milk

- Raw whole milk
- Brie drained cheese
- Fresh yogurt
- Pasteurized milk
- Almond milk

- Fresh lemonade
- Fresh vegetable juice
- Green tea
- Mint tea
- Soy milk
- Tomato juice
- Water with pH level of 7+

Other Foods

- Apple cider vinegar
- Sea salt
- Table salt
- Cold pressed vegetable oils
- Green herbs
- Cinnamon
- Mustard

Foods to eat sparingly

The following foods are known to increase the acidic level in your body, but in order to keep your diet balanced, you should eat very small portions of them per week.

Depending on the current level of your pH, you can determine when and by how much you should start adding these ingredients into your diet. Keep in mind that you are in control of your body and what you feed it, so do not feel that you are deprived of these ingredients. Instead, think of them as something that you should only eat once or twice a month.

Fruit

- Apples
- Mangoes
- Peaches
- Pears
- Figs
- Pineapple
- Dates
- Grapes
- Kiwis
- Oranges
- Papayas
- Strawberries
- Tangerines
- Sweet cherries

Cereal Grain and Breads

- Barley
- Cakes
- Cookies
- Couscous
- Dark bread
- Commercial cereals
- White flour crackers, pasta
- Yeast bread
- Pies
- Semolina
- Sweetened granola
- Wheat
- White bread
- White flour

Dairy

- Aged buttermilk, brie, cheeses, whey, yogurt
- Chocolate milk
- Cooked butter
- Cream
- Dextrogyre yogurt
- Kefir
- Parmesan cheese
- Sweetened yogurt with fruit
- Ultra pasteurized milk

Meat and Fish

Slightly acidifying:

- Bass
- Flounder
- Liver
- Oysters
- Salmon
- Pike
- Sole
- Trout
- Walleye

Acidifying:

- Chicken
- Egg yolk
- Halibut
- Catfish

- Mahi mahi
- Mussels
- Organ meats
- Tuna
- Turkey

Very acidifying:

- Beef
- Carp
- Cold cuts
- Crab
- Lamb
- Lobster
- Herring
- Mackerel
- Pork
- Shrimp
- Whole eggs
- Veal

Other Acidifying Foods and Drinks to Consume Sparingly:

- Brown rice syrup
- Fructose
- Heat pressed vegetable oils
- Honey
- Maple syrup
- Vinegar
- Pickles
- Raw cane sugar
- Artificial sweeteners
- Brown sugar
- Processed foods

- Canned foods
- Capers
- Hydrogenated oils
- Ketchup
- Lard
- Margarine
- Mayonnaise
- Molasses
- Mushrooms
- Pickles
- Pimientos
- White sugar
- Beer
- Black tea
- Carbonated water
- Cocoa
- Coffee
- Commercial juices
- Liquor
- Sodas
- Wine
- Hot chocolate

Chapter 3: Breakfast

Banana Bread Oatmeal

Makes: 1 serving

Ingredients:

- 1/4 cup gluten-free quick oats
- 1 small ripe banana, mashed
- 1/2 cup almond milk
- 2 Tbsp almond butter
- 1 cup fresh blueberries
- 1/4 tsp cinnamon

Directions:

1. Mix together the mashed banana, almond milk and butter, and oats in a saucepan. Place over a medium flame and cook for 2 minutes, stirring frequently.

2. Transfer the oatmeal into a bowl and add the blueberries. Sprinkle the cinnamon on top, mix, and enjoy!

Nutty Breakfast Porridge

Makes: 2 servings

Ingredients:

- 2 cups leftover cooked quinoa
- 2/3 cup vanilla soy milk
- 1 tsp cinnamon
- 1/2 cup nuts or seeds
- 2 tsp dried raisins or dates

Directions:

1. In a saucepan, mix together the quinoa, soy milk, cinnamon, and seeds. Place over a medium flame and stir for 10 minutes.

2. Divide between two bowls and sprinkle the dried raisins or dates on top. Mix and enjoy!

Tofu Scramble

Makes: 2 servings

Ingredients:

- 1/2 lb firm tofu, drained and patted dry
- 1/2 tsp onion powder
- 1/8 tsp turmeric
- 1/4 tsp mustard powder
- 1/8 tsp sea salt
- 1/4 tsp freshly ground black pepper
- 1 Tbsp extra virgin olive oil
- 1/8 cup diced red onion
- 1/2 clove garlic, minced
- 1/2 cup sliced link soy sausage, 1/4 inch rounds
- 2 tsp naturally brewed soy sauce, such as tamari, shoyu, or liquid aminos

Directions:

1. In a bowl, crumble the tofu with a fork. Season with the onion powder, mustard, turmeric, salt, and pepper. Mix and set aside.

2. Place a cast iron skillet over medium flame and heat the olive oil. Sauté the onion and garlic, then season with a dash of sea salt. Sauté for 3 minutes, then stir in the

sausage rounds and cook for an additional 3 minutes, mixing well.

3. Add the tofu and mix well, then add the soy sauce and cook for 3 minutes or until the tofu is browned. Serve warm.

Beans on Toast

Makes: 3 servings

Ingredients:

- 1.5 lb extra firm tofu, drained, patted dry, and sliced into 12 pieces
- 1 1/2 Tbsp naturally brewed soy sauce, such as tamari, shoyu, or liquid aminos
- 1 1/2 cups baked beans
- 6 slices crusty whole grain bread (no yeast)

Directions:

1. Preheat the broiler and prepare a baking sheet by lightly greasing it with olive oil.
2. Place the tofu slices on the prepared baking sheet and broil for 7 minutes. Turn them over with a spatula and broil for an additional 7 minutes, or until golden. Set on a wire rack to cool.
3. Put the baked beans in a saucepan and place over medium flame until warm.
4. Toast the bread slices, then place 2 tofu slices on each toast and spoon the heated beans on top. Serve warm.

Almond Butter Bites

Makes: 4 bars

Ingredients:

- 3/4 cup gluten-free old fashioned oats
- 1/4 cup dried raisins or dates
- 1/2 cup almond butter

Directions:

1. Mix together all three ingredients in a bowl.
2. Press the mixture into a small pan and refrigerate for 2 hours.
3. Slice the mixture into 4 bars and serve chilled. Store in the refrigerator for up to 4 days.

Fresh Watermelon and Spinach Smoothie

Makes: 1 serving

Ingredients:

- 1/4 cup soy or almond milk
- 1/3 cup almond cream, chilled
- 1 cup watermelon, chilled
- 1 Tbsp flax seeds
- 1 cup fresh spinach leaves

Directions:

1. Combine all of the ingredients in a blender. Blend until smooth.
2. Pour into a tall glass and drink at once.

Dandelion Kale Green Smoothie

Makes: 1 serving

Ingredients:

- 1/4 cup dandelion greens
- 1 cup kale leaves
- 1 cucumber
- 1/2 cup celery, diced
- 1/8 cup fresh parsley, minced
- 1/2 cup soy or almond milk

Directions:

1. Blend the dandelion greens, kale, and parsley. Add the cucumber and celery and blend until combined.
2. Add the soy or almond milk and puree until smooth.
3. Pour into a tall glass and serve immediately.

Sweet Potato Smoothie

Makes: 2 servings

Ingredients:

- 2 small sweet potatoes, peeled and cut into cubes
- 1 carrot, peeled and cut into cubes
- 1 cup watermelon, chopped
- 1/4 tsp cinnamon
- 1/8 tsp ground cloves
- 2 cups almond milk

Directions:

1. In a blender, pulse the sweet potato and carrot until combined.
2. Add the watermelon, cinnamon, ground cloves, and almond milk. Blend until smooth.
3. Pour into two tall glasses and serve immediately.

Chapter 4:
Soups and Stews

Creamy Broccoli Soup

Makes: 3 servings

Ingredients:

- 4 cups low sodium vegetable stock
- 1/2 Tbsp extra virgin olive oil
- 2 ribs celery, diced
- 1 small onion, diced
- 2 heads broccoli, chopped into small pieces
- 1 1/2 cups soy milk, plain and unsweetened
- 1/2 container soft or silken tofu, drained
- 1/4 tsp cayenne powder
- 1/2 tsp black pepper, ground
- Sea salt, to taste

Directions:

1. Put the vegetable stock in a saucepan and place over a high flame. Bring to a boil.//
2. Place a skillet over a medium high flame and heat the oil. Sauté the celery and onion with a dash of sea salt until onion is translucent.

3. Add the broccoli to the boiling vegetable stock and cook for 3 minutes. Stir the celery and sautéed onion mixture into the broccoli mixture. Turn off the heat and stir in the soy milk.

4. Put the tofu in a bowl and mash it with your fingers. Add the mashed tofu into the broccoli mixture, then add the cayenne and black peppers. Stir to combine.

5. Blend the soup with a blender or immersion blender and return to the saucepan. Stir and season with salt.

6. Ladle into soup bowls and serve immediately.

Butternut and Celery Soup

Makes: 2 servings

Ingredients:

- 1 celery stalk, sliced into chunks
- 1 butternut squash
- 1 onion, peeled and quartered
- 1 Tbsp olive oil
- 2 cups vegetable stock
- Cinnamon, nutmeg, salt, and pepper, to taste

Directions:

1. Slice the squash and remove the seeds.
2. Preheat the oven to 400 degrees F. Lightly grease a baking sheet.
3. Drizzle the olive oil all over the exposed flesh of the squash and arrange them on the prepared baking sheet, exposed flesh facing upward. Place the celery and onion onto the baking sheet as well.
4. Roast the vegetables for 30 minutes, or until browned.
5. Scoop the soft flesh out of the squash and place into a blender. Add the roasted celery and onion and puree, gradually pouring in the vegetable stock until smooth.
6. Season the soup with cinnamon, nutmeg, salt, and pepper. Ladle into soup bowls and serve immediately.

Miso Stew

Makes: 3 servings

Ingredients:

- 1/2 Tbsp extra virgin olive oil
- 1 small yellow onion, diced
- 1 clove garlic, minced
- 1 small carrot, sliced into 1/4 inch half moons
- 1/2 celery rib, sliced into 1/2 inch half moons
- 1/2 package firm tofu, drained and sliced into 1/2 inch cubes
- 1/4 cup hijiki seaweed, soaked based on package instructions
- 1 cup vegetable stock
- 1 cup filtered water
- 1 cup cooked quinoa
- 1 tsp naturally brewed soy sauce, such as tamari, shoyu, or liquid aminos
- 1 1/2 Tbsp miso paste
- 1/2 tsp freshly grated ginger
- 1 green onion, sliced

Directions:

1. Place a saucepan over a medium flame and heat the oil. Sauté the onion until translucent, then stir in the garlic, carrot, tofu, celery, and seaweed. Sauté until the garlic is fragrant.

2. Add the stock and water, then bring to a simmer. Add the quinoa and soy sauce. Cover and cook for 4 minutes.

3. In a bowl, combine the miso paste and 2 tablespoons of water. Mix well, adding more water to make the miso runny.

4. Turn off the heat under the saucepan and add the ginger to the stew. Stir to mix. Once simmering has completely stopped, add the miso and stir to combine.

5. Sprinkle the green onion on top and serve immediately. Do not reheat.

Tofu and Onion Stew

Makes: 1 serving

Ingredients:

- 1 small onion, sliced
- 1 1/2 cups water
- 2 kale leaves, torn
- 1 bay leaf
- 1 small onion, quartered
- 3/4 cup fresh green beans
- 1 package fresh tofu
- 1/2 Tbsp olive oil
- Sea salt, to taste

Directions:

1. Place the onion in a pan and add 1/2 cup water. Cover and cook for 3 minutes.
2. Add the kale, bay leaf, and remaining water. Cover and let it simmer for 2 minutes, or until kale is wilted.
3. Take out the bay leaf and add the quartered onion and green beans. Cover and let it simmer until tender.
4. Season the stew with salt, then transfer into a bowl. Cover and set aside.

5. Drain and slice the tofu. Place a skillet over a medium flame and heat the oil, then cook the tofu until browned.

6. Place the tofu on top of the onion stew and serve immediately.

Chapter 5: Salads

Greek Lentil Salad

Makes: 3 servings

Ingredients:

Tofu Cheese:

- 1/2 lb extra firm tofu, drained
- 3/4 cup miso paste

Salad:

- 1/2 cup green lentils
- 2 Tbsp extra virgin olive oil
- 1 1/2 Tbsp fresh lemon juice
- 3/4 tsp sea salt
- 1/4 tsp freshly ground black pepper
- 1 Tbsp finely chopped red onion
- 1 small tomato, seeded and diced
- 1/4 cup seeded and diced cucumber
- 1/8 cup finely chopped flat leaf parsley
- 1/2 Tbsp finely chopped fresh oregano

Directions:

1. To make tofu cheese, wrap the tofu using a kitchen towel and squeeze out as much moisture as possible.

2. Spread the miso paste on a plate and put the tofu on top. Spread the rest of the miso all over the tofu. Make sure the entire tofu is smothered in miso paste.

3. Wrap the tofu with a clean cheesecloth and place in a tightly sealed container. Refrigerate from 8 hours to 3 days. The longer, the better.

4. To start preparing the salad, put the lentils on a white plate and remove all pebbles, twigs, and broken lentils. Rinse twice and drain well.

5. Put the lentils in a saucepan and add 1 1/4 cups of water. Place over a medium high flame and bring to a boil.

6. Set the heat to low, cover, and let simmer. Cook for 25 minutes, or until fork tender. Transfer into a large bowl and set aside to cool to room temperature.

7. In a mixing bowl, whisk together the olive oil, lemon juice, salt, and pepper. Add the red onion, tomato, cucumber, parsley, and oregano. Toss in the cooked lentils.

8. Take out the tofu cheese and scrape off the miso. Crumble the tofu cheese on top of the salad, cover, and refrigerate for 3 hours. Serve chilled.

Crunchy Bell Pepper and Cabbage Salad

Makes: 2 servings

Ingredients:

- 1/2 cup red cabbage, thinly sliced
- 1/2 cup green cabbage, thinly sliced
- 1/2 carrot, grated
- 1/2 thinly sliced yellow bell pepper
- 1/2 thinly sliced red bell pepper
- 1/2 thinly sliced orange bell pepper
- 1 Tbsp scallions, chopped
- 1 Tbsp fresh parsley, minced
- 1 Tbsp lemon juice
- 1 Tbsp water
- 1/2 Tbsp extra virgin olive oil or flax seed oil
- 1/2 tsp red chili pepper
- 1/4 tsp apple cider vinegar or liquid aminos

Directions:

1. In a salad bowl, toss together all of the cabbages, followed by the carrot and bell peppers. Toss in the scallions and fresh parsley.

2. Combine the lemon juice, water, oil, chili pepper, and vinegar or aminos. Mix well with a fork, then drizzle all over the salad. Toss to coat.

3. Cover the bowl and chill for 30 minutes, then serve.

Tomato and Avocado Salad

Makes: 2 servings

Ingredients:

- 1/2 small eggplant, diced
- 1 avocado, pitted, peeled, and sliced into cubes
- 1 green chili pepper, seeded and sliced
- 2 tomatoes, thickly sliced
- 1 1/2 cups mung bean sprouts
- 6 leaves organic romaine lettuce, washed and torn
- 1 cup broccoli, lentil, buckwheat, or clover sprouts
- 1 cucumber, peeled and thinly sliced
- 1 carrot, peeled and grated
- 1/2 cup garbanzo beans, sprouted or canned
- 1/2 Tbsp olive oil
- 1 Tbsp silken tofu
- 1 Tbsp lemon juice
- 1/3 Tbsp curry powder

Directions:

1. Lightly steam the eggplant until tender. Place in a bowl and toss in 3/4 of the cubed avocado, followed by the

chili pepper, tomatoes, sprouts, cucumber, carrot, and garbanzo beans.

2. Combine 1/4 of the avocado, olive oil, lemon juice, curry powder, and silken tofu in a blender and blend until smooth. Drizzle the dressing all over the avocado and tomato salad and toss well to coat.

3. Arrange the romaine lettuce on a platter. Pile the avocado and tomato salad on top and serve immediately.

Fresh Spinach and Flax Seed Salad

Makes: 2 servings

Ingredients:

- 1 head spinach
- 3 stalks celery, chopped
- 3/4 cup cauliflower, cut into florets
- 3 radishes, peeled and chopped
- 1 shallot or small red onion, sliced thinly
- 1 red bell pepper, chopped
- 1/4 cup chopped fresh basil
- 2 Tbsp pine nuts
- 1 Tbsp flax seed oil
- 1 Tbsp liquid aminos or apple cider vinegar
- 1 1/4 Tbsp water

Directions:

1. Steam the cauliflower and radishes until fork tender. Place in a bowl and set aside to cool.

2. Mix together the spinach, celery, shallot or red onion, red bell pepper, and basil. Toss in the cooled steamed cauliflower and radish.

3. In a small bowl, combine the liquid aminos or vinegar with the flax seed oil and water. Drizzle all over the spinach salad and toss to coat.

4. Sprinkle the pine nuts on top of the salad and serve immediately.

Festive Vegetable Salad

Makes: 2 servings

Ingredients:

- 2 tomatoes, sliced
- 1 cucumber, sliced and peeled
- 1 red bell pepper, chopped
- 1 green bell pepper, chopped
- 1/2 small red onion, coarsely chopped
- 1 Tbsp diced green chilies
- 1/4 cup fresh cilantro, chopped
- 1 Tbsp lemon juice
- 1/4 Tbsp minced garlic
- Pepper, sea salt, and ground cumin, to taste
- 6 romaine lettuce leaves, washed and torn

Directions:

1. Toss together 1 sliced tomato, cucumber, bell peppers, onion, chilies, and cilantro in a salad bowl. Cover and chill for 30 minutes.

2. Combine the other tomato with the lemon juice, and garlic in a blender. Season with a dash of pepper, sea salt, and ground cumin. Blend until pureed. Adjust seasonings if needed.

3. Drizzle the dressing all over the salad and toss well to coat. Serve immediately.

Rainbow Salad with Soy Cucumber Dressing

Makes: 2 servings

Ingredients:

- 2 beets, grated
- 2 yams, grated
- 2 carrots, grated
- 1 butternut squash or yellow zucchini, grated
- 1 head thinly sliced red cabbage
- 1 red bell pepper, sliced thinly
- 1 thinly sliced yellow bell pepper
- 1 cup mung bean sprouts
- 1/2 cup fresh green peas from the pod
- 1 cucumber, sliced very thinly
- 1 1/2 tsp carrot juice
- 1/2 small onion
- 1/2 red bell pepper
- 1/2 cucumber
- 1/2 cup soy milk
- 1/2 tsp dried basil or 1 tsp fresh basil

- 1 Tbsp apple cider vinegar or liquid aminos

Directions:

1. In a salad bowl, toss together the ingredients, starting with the dark ingredients and ending with the light ingredients. Chill for 15 minutes as you prepare the dressing.

2. In a blender, combine the carrot juice, onion, bell pepper, cucumber, soy milk, basil, and vinegar or liquid aminos. Puree and drizzle all over the salad, then toss to combine. Serve immediately.

Chapter 6: Entrees

Cauliflower and Chickpea Curry

Makes: 3 servings

Ingredients:

- 1 1/2 Tbsp coconut or canola oil
- 1 tsp whole mustard seeds
- 1 small yellow onion, diced
- 2 cloves garlic, minced
- 1 tsp salt
- 1 Tbsp ginger, grated or minced
- 1 1/2 tsp curry powder
- 1/4 tsp garlic powder
- 1 1/2 tsp cumin seeds
- 1/2 tsp ground coriander
- 1/16 tsp ground cloves
- 1/4 tsp ground cinnamon
- 1/8 tsp Asafetida or hing
- 1 green cardamom pod

- 1 cup diced tomatoes, juices reserved

- 4 cups rinsed, stemmed, and chopped fresh spinach

- 1 cup cooked and drained chickpeas

- 1 cup cauliflower, chopped into small pieces

Directions:

1. Place a saucepan over a medium flame and heat the oil. Sauté the mustard seeds until they begin to pop.

2. Stir in the onion and sauté until browned, then stir in the garlic, 1/2 teaspoon of salt, and ginger. Stir until garlic is fragrant.

3. Add the curry and garlic powders, coriander, cumin, cloves, cinnamon, cardamom pod, and Asafetida. Stir in the tomatoes with their juices, then bring to a simmer.

4. Stir in the spinach and cook until wilted. Stir in the chickpeas and cauliflower and add the remaining salt. Stir to combine, then cover and set the heat to low. Cook for 15 minutes.

5. Take out the cardamom pod and serve with warmed whole grain crackers.

Broccoli and Beans

Makes: 4 servings

Ingredients:

- 2 Tbsp extra virgin olive oil
- 2 1/2 cups filtered water
- 1/2 tsp salt
- 1/2 cup organic yellow corn grits
- 1/4 cup diced red onion
- 1 clove garlic, minced
- 1/2 tsp red pepper flakes
- 1 cup cooked and drained pinto beans
- 2 cups broccoli florets
- 1/2 cup low sodium vegetable stock

Directions:

1. Lightly grease a small baking dish with olive oil, then set aside.

2. Place a saucepan over a medium flame and add the water. Stir in 1/4 teaspoons of salt and 1/2 tablespoon of olive oil. Add the corn grits and whisk until boiling.

3. Set the heat to low and continue to stir for about 20 minutes. Once you have cooked the polenta, transfer

into the prepared baking dish and cover with a kitchen towel to keep warm.

4. Place a skillet over a medium high flame and add the remaining olive oil. Sauté the onion until translucent, then add the garlic and remaining salt. Sauté for 1 minute, then add the red pepper flakes.

5. Stir in the beans and broccoli. Mix to combine, then add the vegetable stock and stir. Cover and cook for 5 minutes, then take off the lid and cook for an additional 2 minutes or until the liquid has evaporated.

6. Spoon the polenta into 4 bowls and spoon the beans and broccoli on top. Serve immediately.

Falafel Fritters

Makes: 2 servings

Ingredients:

- 1/8 cup fresh cilantro, chopped
- 1/8 cup fresh parsley, chopped
- 1/2 cup Lima or cranberry beans, soaked overnight, drained, and boiled for 10 minutes
- 3/4 cup chickpeas, rinsed and drained
- 1/2 clove garlic, minced
- 1/2 tsp sea salt
- 1/2 tsp turmeric
- 1/2 tsp cumin
- 1/2 red hot chili pepper, seeds and ribs removed, minced
- 1/8 cup red onion, chopped
- 1/2 Tbsp lime juice
- 1 1/2 Tbsp spelt, whole wheat, or millet flour
- 1 head butter lettuce or savoy cabbage, leaves separated and torn
- 3 cherry tomatoes, quartered
- 1/2 Tbsp toasted sesame seeds

- 1 1/2 Tbsp yellow mustard

- Olive oil

Directions:

1. Combine the cilantro and parsley in the food processor and process until finely chopped.

2. Add the beans, chickpeas, garlic, salt, turmeric, cumin, chili pepper, red onion, lime juice, and flour. Pulse until combined.

3. Preheat the oven to 350 degrees F.

4. Use a tablespoon to scoop the Falafel mixture onto a lightly greased baking sheet. Brush the tops with olive oil, then bake for 10 minutes, or until golden brown.

5. Serve the Falafel fritters with lettuce or cabbage leaves, tomatoes, and sesame seeds. To eat, put a fritter on the center of the leaf and add the tomato, sesame seeds, and mustard. Roll up and enjoy!

Vegan Pad Thai

Makes: 2 servings

Ingredients:

- 1/2 package silken tofu
- 1 1/2 Tbsp almond butter
- 1/6 cup lemon or lime juice
- 1/6 cup liquid aminos
- 1/4 tsp red pepper flakes
- 1/2 small onion, chopped
- 1/2 small bunch green onions, chopped
- 1 cup mixed vegetables, steamed or stir fried
- 4 oz rice noodles
- 1 cup bean sprouts
- 1/3 tsp garlic powder
- 1/2 inch ginger, minced
- 1 Tbsp sesame oil
- Lemon wedges, for serving

Directions:

1. Prepare the rice noodles based on the manufacturer's instructions. Drain and set aside.

2. Press the tofu to get as much moisture out as possible, then slice into 1/2 inch cubes. Set aside.

3. In a bowl, combine the almond butter, lemon or lime juice, liquid aminos, and red pepper flakes. Set aside.

4. Place a wok over a medium flame and heat the sesame oil. Stir fry the garlic and tofu until browned. Stir in the ginger and onions for 2 minutes, then add the vegetables and almond butter mixture. Toss to combine.

5. Stir in the noodles and bean sprouts and toss to combine. Cook until the sauce thickens and everything is heated through. Serve with lemon wedges.

Conclusion

Thank you again for downloading this book!

I hope this book was able to help you learn more about the alkaline diet!

The next step is to put this information to use, and begin improving your health with the help of this dieting technique!

Finally, if you enjoyed this book, please take the time to share your thoughts and post a review on Amazon. It'd be greatly appreciated!

Thank you and good luck!

www.ingramcontent.com/pod-product-compliance
Lightning Source LLC
LaVergne TN
LVHW021739060526
838200LV00052B/3369